Lighting The Fire

A Simple, Basic and Easy-to-Follow
Guide for Beginning Your Health &
Fitness Journey

JORDAN PAUL DUNHAM

ISBN: 1523639431
ISBN-13: 978-1523639434

DEDICATION

I would like to dedicate this book to my parents, Dave & Lisa. Thank you for raising me into the man that I am today. I love you beyond words.

And to Jesus Christ, my Lord and Savior who guides me in all that I do.

DISCLAIMER

This book was written to provide information and motivation to its readers. The concepts, ideas and opinions expressed in this book are intended for educational purposes only. This book is sold with the understanding that both author and publisher are not giving medical advice of any kind, nor is this book intended to replace medical advice. It is also not intended to diagnose, prescribe or treat any disease, condition, illness or injury. It is very important that before starting any nutrition plan or exercise program, including any aspect of this book, you receive full medical clearance from a licensed physician. Author and publisher claim no responsibility to any person or entity for any liabilities, loss, or damage caused or alleged to be caused directly or indirectly as a result of the use, application or interpretation of the material in this book.

CONTENTS

PREFACE

As a junior in high school, I was 5'10" and weighed a whopping 115 pounds. Picture that. I ate like garbage and never worried about my health. I remember being in the school locker room before gym class and hearing my friend joke about how he could see my spine when I took my shirt off to change. I was already self-conscious about how skinny I was, but that comment pushed me over the edge. That day I decided I never wanted to feel like that again. That day was the start of this journey. With eagerness to learn, I began researching online, reading books and taking in all the advice that I could. I got a gym membership in town and began going to health talks and fitness competitions for inspiration.

In the four years that I've been training I've managed to add 55 pounds of lean muscle to my frame, I feel better about myself and I've become passionate about something, that at one point, was a huge negative in my life. This passion has led me to become an entrepreneur in the health and wellness industry and has driven me to travel all over the country to continue learning. In the moment, neither of us knew how much his negative comment would impact my life in such a positive way, but I am extremely thankful to the kid who lit a fire in me that day.

It is my pleasure to share the things that I have learned and experienced with those who are looking to make a change.

INTRODUCTION

First off, allow me to give you a bit of a disclaimer: I am not a personal trainer, nor am I a nutritionist. I am simply a young man on a journey; someone who has become extremely passionate about health and fitness who wants to share his experiences with those who want to listen.

My goal is not to "school" you or portray myself as an expert. My goal is, however, to be the messenger of what I have learned from those who have gone before me. Over the last four years of training I've learned many things from a variety of different people that have helped me to not only transform my body, but my life. I feel that it is my turn to pay it forward. This book, by no means, has all the answers; it is only intended to give you a foundation, and I hope that your desire to learn doesn't end here.

Now, if you are just starting out, I want to say that I'm proud of you. You are taking the initiative to improve yourself and that is something that the majority of the population won't do. *High five!*

The last thing I want to do is overwhelm you. So, for the entirety of this book we'll just stick to the basics.

It seems like almost every day I have people asking me something fitness-related; friends wanting to know what exercises to do, what supplements to take, what to eat, etc. etc. *This* is the reason I am writing this book. I want nothing more than for you to achieve your dream body and your desired state of health. I sincerely hope that after reading this it leaves you feeling inspired and ready to start your journey. In this book, I'll give you the basic tools, but *you*, my friend, have to put those tools to work. I can give you all the information I know, all the tips and tricks I've learned, but it is all worthless if you don't take action.

So, let me start right off the bat with the most important question you'll need to ask yourself before you begin your fitness journey, *"WHY do I want this?"* Sure, working out and eating healthy is awesome and all, but *why* have you decided to pursue this lifestyle? Whether you want to lose weight, gain muscle, or improve your overall health, the question needs to be *"why?"* Is it because you'd like to fit into those jeans you love that have been on the shelf for a few too many years? Get your confidence back? Have more energy to do the things you love?

What is the *why* behind the goal that you are looking to achieve?

Every person reading this is going to have a different goal and a different reason why. It is up to *you* to find the *why* that is specific to you. Before continuing, take a minute and really think about this. I strongly encourage you to jot down your answers on a piece of paper or in the space provided on pages 104 and 105 as a reference for you to look back on regularly. These answers alone will essentially be your engine, the very thing that keeps you going.

With that being said, I can promise you that this journey will get tough. You WILL want to quit. But when the tough times come, and believe me they will, you will be ready.

"When you embark on this journey you must know that it's gonna go down before it comes up, and when it comes up it's gonna go so much higher than you have ever been."

-Greg Plitt: American fitness model and former Army Ranger

Thus far, I can honestly say that being in the gym has made me a better man in all areas of my life. My fellow gym-rats can vouch for me on that. Every day it teaches valuable life lessons such as discipline, patience, persistence, perseverance, humility, and so many more. It takes a lot of hard work to transform the human body, and the traits that you will acquire from doing so will carry over to your every day life. I've never met someone who has told me that they regret getting into fitness.

You've made one of the best decisions you will ever make, and I am truly excited for you! Let's go.

1 THE PERKS OF A LIFESTYLE CHANGE

"A lifestyle change begins with a vision and a single step."

-Jeff Galloway: Former member of the 1972 U.S. Olympic team

In my opinion, and the opinion of health professionals, every physically abled person should be exercising on a daily basis. There are many great things that this lifestyle can offer, but for the sake of keeping this book short, I'll only focus on the three that I believe to be the most fun.

1. **Physical improvements** will happen when we commit to going to the gym and following a good food plan. Muscle growth, fat loss, regaining higher energy levels and boosting our overall health are some of the most obvious benefits. These are the things that everyone seems to strive for, but are only the beginning to a long list of benefits.

2. The next benefit is **mental strength**. Think about the simple concept of working on something and putting extreme amounts of effort into that project, piece of artwork, etc. There is a huge amount of satisfaction in a job well-done, correct? Now, think about doing that with your body. Your physical-being is the very thing that you see and feel every single day.

How will you feel when you're seeing your hard work unfold right before your eyes? What do you think that will do for your confidence? Personally, being someone who often lacked self-esteem and confidence, it has been life changing.

I use the lessons that I learn in the gym in every area of my life, and there is not a doubt that I'm a better son, brother, friend, uncle, boyfriend and leader because of it. I don't say these things to impress you or boast about myself, I say them to impress *upon* you that fitness can drastically change a person for the better. All of this sounds great, but again, I feel that there is one more area that trumps all others.

3. **Spirituality** probably isn't the first thing that most people think of when they consider starting a journey towards being fit and healthy, and I

am definitely guilty of that. Over the last year or so, I have finally seen how the two go hand-in-hand.

I want to live for my Creator and make Him proud by taking care of the body He has blessed me with. After all, it really is the only place that I have to live.

We need to treat our bodies like the temples that He intended them to be. This has been monumental for my mind set, my goals, and my overall progress. For me, this is becoming the most fulfilling part of this lifestyle and my hope for you (whatever your faith may be) is that it becomes the centerpiece for your journey as well.

2 YOU ARE WHAT YOU EAT. DON'T BE FAST, CHEAP, EASY AND FAKE

"We now know that optimal nutrition is the key to long-term good health."

-Dr. Myron Wentz: Double PhD, Microbiologist, Immunologist, Founder of Usana Health Sciences and Sanoviv Medical Institute

I often find that many people put their training before their nutrition, which is easily the biggest mistake one can make. Hey, I've been guilty of it too, but what I've come to realize is that going to the gym for sixty minutes is indeed very important, but it's what you're doing with the other 23 hours that is even more crucial. Don't worry, it is perfectly normal to not have a clue what you're doing or where to begin when it comes to proper nutrition.

Have you ever found yourself in the middle of the grocery store, feeling like you're in another world? Ever become so overwhelmed that you just say, "screw it" and settle for the "fat-free" and "low calorie" frozen food section? That was me! I had no idea what I was doing when I first started and it didn't help that food labels claimed to be "healthy." I figured that if the label said so, it had to be true, right? Not entirely.

Look, I know that it's hard. I know that it's not what you're used to and that you may feel overwhelmed at times. I've felt the same way, but I can assure you that it doesn't have to be as stressful as most of us make it.

Eating healthy and having a decent food plan is actually quite simple. In this chapter I'll cover 6 common questions and give you the answers you'll need to know.

1. Why is nutrition so important?
2. What are macronutrients and micronutrients?
3. What is the glycemic index and glycemic roller coaster?
4. What does a complete and healthy meal consist of?
5. What part of the grocery store should I shop in?
6. Is there a convenient way to get a complete and balanced meal on-the-go?

1. Why is nutrition so important?

I cannot stress enough how important nutrition is for achieving your desired physique, but more importantly, an optimally healthy lifestyle. Think of the foods that you eat like putting gas in your car. No gas means you can't go anywhere and your car can't serve its purpose. I don't know about you, but I've had times where I get in my car and realize that the gas tank is on E, the low fuel light is blinking at me and I'm worrying if I can even make it to the gas station to fill up!

The importance of gas for your car is the same as nutrients for your body. We need fuel to function, and we most definitely need a higher grade of fuel to perform and function optimally. When we are consistently eating the SAD diet (standard American diet) of junky, fast, cheap, and fake foods that hold zero nutritional value, we are depriving our bodies of the nutrients they desperately need.

You wouldn't put windshield washer fluid in your gas tank, would you? No, of course not, because it would damage your car. The same is true for our mouths and the low quality foods that we're eating. We are damaging our bodies and every time we take a bite out of that fast-food cheeseburger, we're distancing ourselves from our goals and we're also allowing disease to slowly creep in. Our bodies are machines, and they were designed to take a certain type of fuel. So please, don't settle for the junk just because it's convenient.

2. What are Macronutrients and Micronutrients?

Macronutrients provide calories and are the nutrients that most of us are familiar with. These are carbohydrates, proteins and fats.

Carbohydrates:

-Provides fuel during exercise and fuel for the central nervous system

-Spares protein to preserve muscle during exercise

Protein:

-Necessary for the structure, function, and regulation of the body's tissues and organs

-Used for repairing and building muscle

Fats:

-Reserves energy

-Protects vital organs

-Transfers fat-soluble vitamins

Micronutrients are the nutrients required to manage physiological functions. These are vitamins, minerals and antioxidants that are essential for optimal health.

Vitamins:

-Allows the body to break down and use the basic elements and energy that food provides

Minerals:

-Contains essential nutrients we need to survive and carry out daily functions

-Helps antioxidants do their job

<u>Antioxidants:</u>

-Stops the oxidation process that is continuously happening inside and outside of the body

3. What is the glycemic index and glycemic roller coaster?

The **Glycemic Index** was created by a man named Dr. David Jenkins who is a professor in the department of Nutritional Sciences at the University of Toronto, Canada. His first writings about the Glycemic Index appeared in the *American Journal of Nutrition* in 1981 and he has since authored at least 15 more clinical studies on this topic.

Jenkins came up with this chart to better describe how fast carbohydrates are absorbed into the bloodstream. Based on the results, he labeled the carbs as either *low glycemic* or *high glycemic*. Low, (55 and under) being a healthy range, and high, (70 and above) being an unhealthy range. High-glycemic foods are refined carbohydrates that have high amounts of sugar and a high sugar-conversion rate. A few examples of high-glycemic foods are pasta, white rice, most breads and any other foods that are made with refined white flour.

The Glycemic Index can be used for having a better understanding of weight loss and also disease prevention. In short, a basic understanding of how this applies to your overall health is this: When you eat a carbohydrate, it is digested and absorbed into the blood stream. If that carbohydrate is *high-glycemic,* it will spike the blood sugar at a rapid speed and the body will release a hormone called insulin. Insulin is a fat storage hormone. Did you catch that? Insulin is a **fat** storage hormone.

When insulin is consistently spiked, weight gain will become a side effect. Excessive weight gain can lead to Type 2 diabetes, heart disease and other problems. If we can learn to control our insulin levels with the foods we eat, we can have a better grasp on not only gaining those unwanted pounds, but we can also steer away from other health complications associated with poor eating habits.

Glycemic Index Chart

Low GI < 55		Moderate GI 55-70		High GI > 70	
Soy Beans	16	Rice Noodles	58	White Bread	70
Cashew Nuts	22	Honey	61	Saltine Crackers	74
Kidney Beans	26	Gluten Free Pancakes	61	Puffed White Rice	74
Barley	29	Coca Cola	63	French Fries	75
Lentils	34	White Flour Spaghetti	65	Total Cereal	76
Raw Carrots	35	McDonald's Hamburger	66	Gatorade	78
Soy Milk	36	Popcorn	66	White Flour Pancakes	80
Raw Apple	36	McDonald's McChicken	66	Jelly Beans	80
Strawberries	40	Fruit Syrup Diluted	66	Special K	84
Dates	42	Corn Meal	68	Pretzels	84
Oranges	43	Gnocchi Pasta	68	Instant Boil Rice	87
Sweet Potato	44	Bagel	69	Fruit Bars	90
Peaches	47			Rice Cracker	91
Corn Tortilla	48			Kellogs Corn Flakes	93
Whole Wheat Spaghetti	50			Potato Bread	101
Raw Banana	53			Jasmine Rice	109
Long Grain Brown Rice	55				
Sweet Corn	55				

Although my goals don't include losing weight, they do however include being as healthy as possible. The same may be true for you, and if so, don't brush this off just because you aren't looking to lose weight. Aim for optimal health no matter how "in shape" your physique looks. This is why I take advantage of the glycemic index [on the previous page] and use it as a resource for eating low-glycemic meals. If you don't see a certain food on the GI chart, you can *Google* any food's GI number.

If you *are* looking to lose weight; learning the glycemic index will help you tremendously. Apply these things into your lifestyle and you will be on the path to optimal health and fitness.

The **Glycemic Roller coaster** is exactly what it sounds like; a scary ride with all kinds of twists, turns and crazy drops that will turn your stomach upside down. Much like a normal roller coaster that you will find at the big amusement parks, the glycemic roller coaster also has plenty of ups and downs. Except with this coaster, you're not in a little car speeding down the rails. Instead, it's your insulin and blood sugar levels that have the "joy" of experiencing the wild ride.

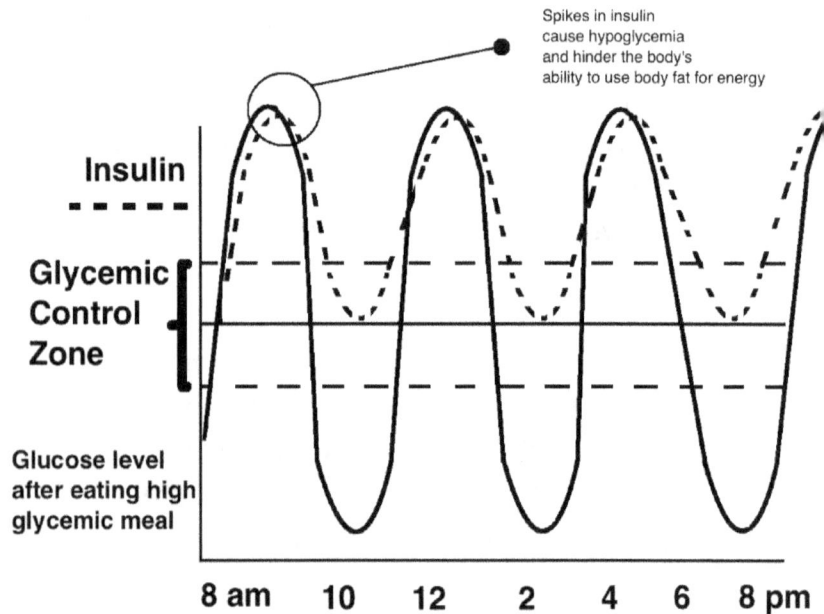

Spikes in insulin cause hypoglycemia and hinder the body's ability to use body fat for energy

Insulin

Glycemic Control Zone

Glucose level after eating high glycemic meal

8 am   10   12   2   4   6   8 pm

All jokes aside, the glycemic roller coaster is something that most of us are riding all throughout the day and this is definitely not good. As you can see in the picture above; from the time we wake up 'til the time we go to bed, we're eating foods that are sending our blood sugar levels sky high and after about an hour they come crashing back down.

So, naturally, what do we do when these levels plummet? We go right back to the cupboard for more high glycemic foods because we feel groggy, tired and extremely hungry. The rollercoaster also affects our cravings. We crave junk food and refined carbohydrates because they satisfy our hunger very quickly. This doesn't make us bad people, it's just our body's natural response, telling us that we need to get our blood sugar back up.

-Did you know that refined carbohydrates are said to be 10 times **more** addictive than crack-cocaine? I heard this statistic in a documentary (*Fed Up*) and it blew my mind. We are literally, to a certain degree, addicted to junk food and it has very quickly become an epidemic.

After we eat the high glycemic food we've been craving, our energy is boosted back up, only for it to come crashing down again. This constant up and down process is reoccurring week after week, month after month and will eventually turn into a lifetime if we don't become aware of it.

The picture below is what we should be striving for. Low-glycemic foods keep the blood sugar and insulin levels in a controlled range and allow us to have consistent energy through-out the day.

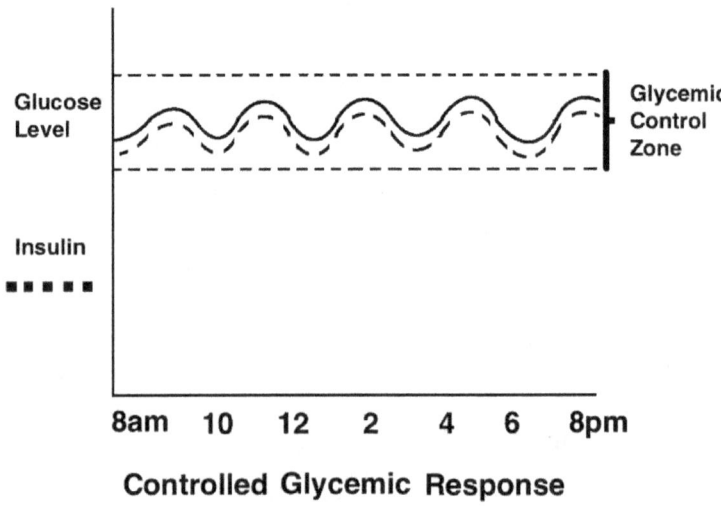

Controlled Glycemic Response

You can avoid riding the glycemic roller coaster and all of the problems that come with it by using the tips you will learn in the next section.

4. What does a complete and healthy meal consist of?

Earlier, I briefly touched on the importance of proper nutrition and what we should *not* be putting into our bodies, so it begs the question of what we *should* be putting into our bodies.

I regularly attend local health events, and my friend, Eric, is often times the main speaker. He has his master's in Human Performance, in addition to many other impressive credentials. He is a huge believer in eating whole and real foods that come from the earth, and I absolutely agree with him. God didn't put fruits, vegetables and certain animals on this planet to make it look pretty. He put them here for a reason and that reason is to consume them in order to survive and stay healthy.

Dr. Steve is another man who regularly

speaks at events in my hometown. He always asks this question, "Have you ever seen a donut bush?" Obviously that's a ridiculous question because of course you haven't seen a donut bush! Get the point?

A good rule of thumb: If it comes from the earth, eat it. If it doesn't, don't. This rule isn't always the end-all, but for the most part it is a helpful reminder.

-Again, this book is meant to be very basic and inspire you to continue learning about these things. For that reason, I am not going to lay out a full meal plan. My hope is that you can take this information and come up with a food plan that best fits your personal preferences and goals.

So what does a healthy meal consist of? First off, your meals need to be balanced. Remember how we talked about what macronutrients are? Each meal needs to have low glycemic carbohydrates, proteins and fats. Every macronutrient serves a unique purpose and is most efficient when in unison with the others.

Try not to eat meals that are missing one or more of the macronutrients the body needs. An example of one of my favorite meals consists of chicken breast (protein), sweet Potato fries from scratch (Low-glycemic carbs), avocado (healthy fats), and broccoli (vitamins, minerals and antioxidants). This is a balanced meal and what each of them should look like.

Don't like Chicken? Swap it out for some fish or eggs etc. You can do the same with carbs and fats. Mix and match foods that you like, but make sure they are still whole and real foods that will keep your meals balanced. No mixing in pop-tarts just because the label says they have carbs, proteins and fats. Not all nutrients are created equal!

Think of food as information. When you are eating *real* food, your body knows what to do with the information its been given and which direction to go. A hundred calories of cake gives very different information than a hundred calories of broccoli. Does this mean that you can never have a piece of cake or go out to eat with friends? No, of course not. Those are celebration foods. Just make sure you're not celebrating every day! I personally really like to use the 80/20 rule: 80% healthy food, 20% celebration food.

In the next section you can find my actual grocery list and all of the foods that I mix and match to make balanced meals.

5. What section of the grocery store should I shop in?

Like I mentioned earlier, I never knew what to look for when I went to the grocery store. It was always a set back for me. Early on, a friend of mine told me to focus on shopping on the outside perimeter of the store, and his advice made all the difference. I never realized it until he said it, but almost every grocery store keeps all of the fresh vegetables, lean meats and low-glycemic carb sources on the perimeter. This isn't *always* the case, but chances are if it's in the middle of the store, it's probably boxed and highly processed. This is a good rule of thumb that helps me!

My personal grocery list: (Example)

Protein

-Chicken Breasts

-Steak

-Ground Beef

-Ground Turkey

-Eggs

-Whey meal replacement shake

Low-Glycemic Carbs

-Sweet Potatoes

-Oats

-Quinoa (similar to rice)

-Long grain brown rice

-Vegetables

Low-Glycemic Snacks

-Bananas

-Apples

-Dates

-Raisins

-Raspberries

-Nuts

Fats

-Avocados

-Nuts

-Grape Seed Oil (used for cooking)

Suggestion: Look online or on Pinterest for healthy whole-food recipes!

6. Is there a way to get a complete and balanced meal "on-the-go"?

One of my training partners, Ryan, has always been really good at staying consistent with his meal prep. He picks a day out of each week and cooks all of his meals in bulk so they are ready in advance. This is definitely the most effective way that I've found, but it's still easy to slip up and fall behind at times.

For this reason and a few others, I get

really excited about meal replacement shakes. Not protein shakes; **meal replacement** shakes. There is a huge difference and it goes back to having the balance of nutrients that I mentioned before. The convenience of having a complete and healthy meal that I can mix up, practically anywhere, has been game changing for me.

My buddies and I took a day-trip to a state park over the summer. We are all into fitness and love the lifestyle, but when you are out in the middle of nowhere it's kind of difficult to whip up some food and have a decent meal. They went hungry for most of the day, but I was able to stay full and not miss a meal because I had my shakes with me.

I'm sure you won't always be out in the middle of nowhere with nothing to eat, but what about traveling? Airport food is off-the-charts expensive. What about when you're in a work meeting? Or your boss tells you that you can't take a lunch break because you're too busy? Still having the option to get in a fast and healthy meal is majorly important.

In the next chapter I'll explain in detail exactly what you should look for when choosing the right supplements. Meal replacement shakes are no exception when it comes to quality and should meet a certain criteria.

In short, to answer the question, "is there a complete and balanced meal option for on-the-go circumstances?" The answer is YES.

3 FILLING THE GAPS

"I believe that you can, by taking some simple and inexpensive measures, lead a longer life and extend your years of well-being. My most important recommendation is that you take vitamins every day in optimum amounts to supplement the vitamins that you receive in your food."

-Dr. Linus Pauling: American chemist, biochemist, two-time Nobel Prize winner and rated the 16th most important scientist in history

When I first got into training I had no idea about supplementation whatsoever. I, like many others, tried many kinds of "fad" supplements thinking that it was going to be the "magic pill" that would speed everything up. In my experience that wasn't the case. I feel that this topic is often misunderstood and leads to people avoiding supplementation altogether, which is not good.

Supplements are crucial in achieving optimal health and when we use the right ones they can only help us progress. *But*, which ones are good for us, and which ones aren't? What I've learned is that all supplements are not created equal. Unfortunately, the supplement industry is *not* regulated.

Companies are putting whatever they want into their products and no one is holding them accountable. Studies have shown that multiple companies have failed third party testing due to contaminants in their products such as lead, traces of petroleum oil and other foul ingredients.

I can imagine that you are reading this and thinking to yourself "How can he say these things, yet still say that supplements are necessary?" Well friends, the good news is that there are a few excellent companies out there that happen to voluntarily hold themselves to a much higher standard.

So why are supplements so important? The answer is quite simple, but before we get into that let's backtrack just a tad. We all know that our bodies need nutrients to stay alive, correct? We need all kinds of vitamins and minerals to keep our cells healthy, which in turn keep *us* healthy. This isn't news to any of us. So, why do we continue to be so severely nutrient deficient as a population? [see chart on the next page]

Percentage of U.S. population NOT meeting the RDA levels of nutrients

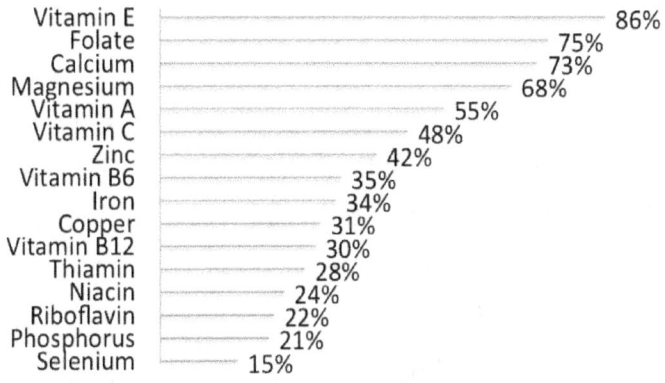

Source: United States Department of Agriculture (2009)

The best way to get the essential nutrients and antioxidants that we need is through fruits and vegetables. This wasn't a problem back when great grandma and grandpa were kids, but the times have changed and continue to change. Foods are no longer grown the way they once were, soil isn't as rich and full of minerals as it used to be and we're using more chemicals than we ever have before. Do a quick *Google* search and see for yourself. This is scary stuff.

One quick example to give you an idea of what I'm talking about is Vitamin E. Did you know that you would have to eat 27 pounds of spinach *every day* just to get the recommended amounts that we need? That is for the RDA levels, I'm not even talking about optimal levels. (Achieving RDA levels are equivalent to aiming for a D- in math class.) Also, that is only one vitamin. Imagine trying to do that for every single one of them. I think it's safe to say that you're probably not eating three 9-pound salads every day. I'm definitely not!

This is why I choose to supplement. Am I against eating fruits and vegetables? Absolutely NOT. Notice how I say supplement, not substitute. That brings us back to our original question, "Why are supplements so important?" They are important and absolutely necessary for the simple fact that we just cannot get all of the nutrients that we need from our food alone. Supplements help us to fill the gaps that we may be missing. More nutrients equals better health and better health equals better results in the gym. It's an upward cycle towards being healthy and it all starts with our cells.

When looking for the right brand of supplements to use, you'll need to make sure that you can check off some often overlooked, yet *very* important credentials.

1. Does the company and its products have a great reputation? Not only based on the opinions of its consumers, but more importantly on the third party testing done by professionals. If the answer is no, then there is obviously a good reason for that. Stay away from that company.

- A great tool to use is a book called "NutriSearch: Comparative Guide to Nutritional Supplements" by Lyle McWilliams

-In his book, Lyle McWilliams compares over 1,500 companies and rates them between one and five stars based on strict qualifications.

2. Are their products made in house? In other words, does the company make their own products in their own facility? Again, if the answer is no, stay away.

3. Is the facility FDA registered? Like I said earlier on, the supplement industry is NOT regulated. This means that no one is holding these companies accountable for what is going into their products. I highly recommend finding a company that voluntarily adheres to the regulations set by the FDA. To go a step further, like I did, I recommend finding a brand that adheres to pharmaceutical regulations. This is the highest and purest quality of supplements that you will find.

4. Does the company have a potency guarantee? This guarantees that what is on the label, is EXACTLY what is in the bottle. Unfortunately, this is not the case for the majority of supplements, but it is a crucial credential that you need to look for to avoid putting any extra junk in your system that may be in the company's product.

5. Finally, the simplest question is, **does the product actually work?** The worst thing is to invest into something and have it do nothing. We've all had our fair share of bad investments and we all know how much it stinks. Search for testimonies from real people who have had real results. Now, I will say that supplements are very different than pharmaceutical drugs. It will take at least a few months to notice a difference in the way you feel, but the difference is that it is addressing the roots and not just covering up the symptoms. So talk around, find a company that passes these five benchmarks, attend some events to learn from experts and give that brand a fair shot for at least 3-6 months. You will be very happy that you did!

Note: I highly recommend that everyone uses *at least,* a high quality multi-vitamin and a high quality fish oil supplement.

An easy experiment you can do to test to see if your multivitamins are high quality is through an apple test. Cut an apple in fourths and place one of the pieces in a cup of water. (The oxidation that happens to a sliced apple is similar to that of what happens to our cells in our bodies.) Take the recommended dosage of your multivitamin and place them in the water with the apple.

Let them sit for 48 hours. If your apple is still crisp and it looks the same as before-congratulations! You've found yourself a quality supplement. If it doesn't look the same then toss that thing in the trash along with the vitamins you did the test with!

4 WE'RE JUST GETTING WARMED UP

"One of the basic ways to avoid injury is to always make sure to stretch and warm up your body. This will loosen up your muscles, which will help to avoid common strain injuries."

-Laurieann Gibson: Former dance choreographer for Michael Jackson, Beyonce and Alicia Keys

Many of us who go to the gym often times skip warming up properly. We're anxious to get in there and kill our workouts,

I get it. But what we're skipping is one of the most important parts of training. Preventing injury is the very thing that's going to keep us in the game. If you're injured, there are no results to be made. This is a lifestyle and we're in it for the long haul, right? So, we need to be treating it as such.

Looking back, it occurred to me that almost all of my past injuries or times where I've felt soreness (not the good kind) could be traced back to not taking care of the little things. This can include warming up properly and stretching after a workout. Please learn from my mistakes and implement the things you will learn in this chapter into your routine and make a habit of it.

Why is warming up before a workout so important?

When I was a kid my siblings and I would always jump on the trampoline. At the end of every fall season our parents said that it needed to be taken down because the cold weather could damage the mat. Have you ever jumped on a trampoline when it's cold outside? If you have, then you've probably noticed that during the first few bounces the mat feels like it could tear right down the middle. The elasticity in the mat is cold and stiff until you walk around on it and stretch it out first.

The same is true for our joints, muscles, tendons and ligaments. If you go straight into heavy resistance training or set out for a long run before warming up properly you are putting yourself in a very vulnerable position; much like the trampoline that's been sitting in the cold. In order to avoid possible injuries, we have to get ourselves warmed up before we start our training.

The most effective way I've found to do this is to warm up through the exercise that you're about to do. It is important that we try to avoid doing long static-stretches (see definition: pg. 101) before we warm up.

Personally, I try my best to avoid stretching while my muscles are still "cold." I would highly suggest you do as well. Along with the trampoline analogy, this would also be similar to putting a rubber band in the freezer and then trying to stretch it to it's full potential. As you probably already know, the rubber band is going to snap very quickly. Please note, "warming up" and stretching are not the same thing.

To keep this basic and easy to understand, I'll use weightlifting as an example.

A quick example of a proper warm up:

If you are going to bench press, squat, deadlift etc. etc., aim for 2-3 warm up sets before you get into your heavier sets. Start your first warm up set with around 50% of your "working set" (see definition: pg. 102) capability. For your second set do 60%, and your third, 70%. Now you're warmed up and ready for those heavier sets, just make sure that you don't burn yourself out on your warm ups. 8-10 reps per set is plenty.

Remember, this philosophy is not only for weightlifting, it can be applied with any type of training. If you're going for a run, begin by walking at a quick pace for 10 minutes. If you're doing hill sprints, jog up and down the hill a few times first. If you're lifting weights, follow the strategy on the previous page.

These are obviously very vague examples, but they all bring me back to my main point - always warm up through the movements in which you are about to perform.

After we have properly warmed up and completed our training for the day, we can do some basic stretching. You'll find that stretching after you work out will reduce soreness the next day and it is also a great way to lower the risk of injury.

I recommend looking online, to find

several different stretches and techniques.

5 THE NUTS & BOLTS OF FITNESS

"Training gives us an outlet for suppressed energies created by stress and thus tone the spirit just as exercise conditions the body."

-Arnold Schwarzenegger: Former professional bodybuilder and 7X Mr. Olympia winner

So far we've talked about the benefits of a healthy lifestyle, the importance of nutrition, supplementation and why we should properly warm-up before training. All of these topics have led us to the next piece in the puzzle: Exercising.

Like I mentioned earlier, every physically-abled person should be exercising on a daily basis. If you're reading this book, I'm assuming that you've already made the decision to take this seriously. So, where should you start?

Truthfully, starting out is actually pretty simple if you stick with the basics. In this chapter, I'll break down 3 different types of exercising that I believe will serve you very well: **strength training**, **high intensity interval training** and **yoga**.

With hard work and dedication, these three examples have helped play a part in the results that I've achieved. I believe that the same can be true for you. No matter what your goals are, the things you will learn in this chapter can help you reach them. The only variable is how much effort *you* are willing to put in.

1. Strength Training

Wikipedia's definition says: "Strength training is a type of physical exercise specializing in the use of resistance to induce muscular contraction which builds strength, anaerobic endurance, and size of skeletal muscles."

This includes weight lifting, body weight exercises and resistance bands or machines.

The definition goes on to say: "When properly performed, strength training can provide significant functional benefits and improvement in overall health and well-being."

When people think of strength training, the impression they might have is often a pre-conceived idea that the only people who exercise this way are "meat heads" and jocks. Am I right? From conversations I've had, I've found that this is one of the biggest reasons why people don't pursue it. They feel that they don't fit the part, or they don't want to get "too big." They brush it off as something that isn't for them and totally miss out on every reason why it's exactly what they need. You see, strength training isn't only for bodybuilders, football players, etc. etc. It can truly benefit everyone. And yes, ladies, I'm talking to you too!

So, why should you consider starting a strength training program? Like I mentioned briefly in chapter 1, there are quite a few benefits from exercising. Let's go further into detail on how strength training, in specific, can be beneficial for you. I've broken this section down into 5 reasons why I highly recommend it.

You can expect:

1. A more effective way to get in shape
2. The most effective way to gain muscle mass
3. Better heart health
4. A longer life expectancy
5. An increase in bone strength

(1) A more effective way to get in shape

A common misconception many people have is that cardio makes you lose fat, and strength training makes you gain muscle. It's as simple as that, right?

Both of these statements may be true. However, when you're walking on the treadmill for 30 minutes everyday, you *are* burning calories and losing fat, *but* you're also losing precious muscle mass along with it. A steady-pace cardio approach, at best, will only dwindle you down to a smaller version of your current physique. Yes, you'll lose weight but this approach will deny you the opportunity to look "toned" and have an "in-shape" physique.

On the flip side of the coin, you have the option to choose strength training as the majority of your time spent while working out. Not only will you be losing fat, but you will also be maintaining and/or building more muscle mass along the way. This will lead to a much better transformation and leave you feeling more satisfied with your results.

One thing that must be addressed about this topic, is that women often avoid strength training and lifting heavy weights (more than 10-20 pounds) because they are afraid of looking "manly" or "too buff." Ladies, I hate to break it to you, but these assumptions are far from the truth. Believe me when I say that it is extremely difficult to gain large amounts of muscle mass and it takes years of intentional focus.

Since women do not produce testosterone, there is no possible way that you will *accidentally* get "too big." Lifting heavy weights will, however, allow for greater fat-loss and will provide more muscle definition once body fat is reduced. This goes for men too, don't be worried about getting too big on *accident*. It won't happen.

So, whether you are male or female, do

not avoid strength training!

(2) The best way to gain muscle mass

We've talked a lot about fat-loss so far, but this section is specifically written for those whose goals are to gain muscle mass.

In the preface of this book I shared a little bit about my background in training and *why* I decided to pursue health and fitness. As you have already read, I was the skinny kid who lacked confidence and desperately wanted to feel good about himself.

If this is where you're at, I can especially relate to you. Implement the concepts in this book, and like myself, you may have found just what you've been looking for.

As I mentioned in the last section, building muscle is extremely difficult and takes years of hard work and patience. But that's not to say you can't make great gains in the beginning. Actually, it is within your first year that you will see the most gain in muscle mass and overall size.

Since my body wasn't used to the heavy weight training when I first began, it was forced to add more muscle and become stronger. By the end of my first year of consistent training and good nutrition, I had already put on about 25 pounds. This may not seem like much, but the changes that an additional 25 pounds of muscle will make are drastic.

However, everyone is different, and your results may look different than mine or someone else's. Don't worry about comparing yourself to the person next to you. Walk your own walk, stay consistent and the results will come.

In order to increase muscle mass, you need to be progressively over-loading your muscles during training. This means that you are using resistance (strength training) to break down the muscle fibers. With consistent training, progression and proper form, the muscle will be forced to grow larger over time. This happens because the muscle fibers will repair themselves, grow back stronger and become bigger.

It is simply a survival mechanism that our bodies have. When we are progressively overloading the muscle with heavy resistance, it's natural defense is to become bigger and stronger in order to handle the new type of stress that training provides.

For this reason, it is especially important to continue progressing (adding more weight/resistance), because once our bodies adapt to the stress, our muscles have no reason to keep growing.

So, why is strength training the best way to gain muscle mass? The name itself is a good indicator, but I'll give you a better explanation. In order to get bigger, we must first become stronger. Ronnie Coleman said it best, "Everybody wants be a bodybuilder but nobody wants to lift no heavy weights."

The heavier we lift and the stronger we become, the deeper we will break down the fibers that our muscles are made of. This is what causes growth. I've found that strength training is the best way to keep track of your strength progression, which will lead to more muscle mass. You can never become too strong for the weight room. There will always be bigger and heavier weights waiting for you.

If muscle growth is your goal, strength training is your answer.

(3) Better heart health

Researchers with the University of Michigan did a test on people who strength trained three times per week for two months. They found that it reduced their diastolic blood pressure by 8 points on average, which could bring down the chances of having a stroke by 40% and 15% for a heart attack.

(4) A longer life expectancy

A study done by researchers from the University of South Carolina came to the conclusion that overall body strength can lower the risk of death from heart disease and cancer. A different set of scientists determined that being strong can help us live well into our 80's without developing a major disease.

(5) An increase in bone strength

Here is what the Harvard Medical Institute says about bone strength and its correlation with strength training in a recent article:

> Most of us know that strength training (with free weights, weight machines, or resistance bands) can help build and maintain muscle mass and strength. What many of us don't know is that strong muscles lead to strong bones. And strong bones can help minimize the risk of fractures due to osteoporosis.
>
> Osteoporosis should be a concern for all of us. An estimated eight million women and two million men in the United States have osteoporosis. It is

now responsible for more than two million fractures each year, and experts expect that number will rise. Hip fractures are usually the most serious. Six out of 10 people who break a hip never fully regain their former level of independence. Even walking across a room without help may become impossible.

Numerous studies have shown that strength training can play a role in slowing bone loss, and several show it can even build bone. This is tremendously useful to help offset age-related declines in bone mass. Activities that put stress on bones can nudge bone-forming cells into action. That stress comes from the tugging and pushing on bone that occur during strength training (as well as weight-bearing aerobic exercises like walking or running). The result is stronger, denser bones.

Like Benjamin Franklin once said, "An ounce of prevention is worth a pound of cure." Let's take care of ourselves now so we can thank ourselves later.

Switching gears

We've covered the benefits of strength training and we've debunked a few popular myths along the way. Now that we're clear on how effective strength training is for both fat-loss *and* muscle growth, for both men *and* women, let's dive into some important things you need to know once you've decided to start a program.

- The gym isn't as scary as you may think
- Proper form is more important than quick strength gains
- Practice gym etiquette

The gym isn't as scary as you think

Before I signed up with my first gym, I worked out in my garage with my older brother, Luke. During one of our workouts he started talking about getting a gym membership, and I remember telling him that he'd be going by himself if he did such a thing. I was so intimidated by the thought of working out around people who were so much further along than I was. I was self conscious about how I looked and felt that people would judge me. So, I stayed comfortable in my little one-car garage and put a cap on my potential.

Friends, this is what we call a *limiting belief*. I was holding myself back because I had it built up in my head that the gym was an intimidating and scary place.

Luke ended up getting a gym membership, and after some convincing, I finally decided I would too. But it didn't end there - I would only go at 6 a.m. because the place was empty... Pathetic, I know!

I say this because maybe you're feeling the same way. Maybe you're on the fence about joining your local gym. Well, I want to push you off that dang fence (in the nicest way possible, of course) so you can finally realize what I realized. The gym is *not* as scary as you think!

To make this step even less intimidating, find someone you know who already has a gym membership. Ask them if you can tag along to their gym and have them show you around. If no one comes to mind, most gyms will give you a tour of their facility before you sign on the dotted line. As a result, there is a good chance you will begin to feel more comfortable with joining a gym.

When I decided to stop succumbing to my fears, I started tapping into my potential. The people who I assumed would be judging me soon became great friends and before long, they were offering to teach me everything they knew. Why? Because my assumptions were incorrect from the start.

If you resonate at all with how I once felt, I urge you to take the leap. You will soon find out for yourself that joining a gym is a fantastic investment.

Proper form is more important than quick strength gains

There is a certain way that each exercise is meant to be executed. This is called having proper form. I see people every day who are slapping on more and more weight and their form gets progressively worse with each rep.

Honestly, it hurts to watch.

We should never be sacrificing our form and flailing around like a chicken with its head cut off just so we can say that we lifted more weight. Yes, the goal may be to get stronger, but never with the exception of doing it the wrong way. This may boost our egos, but it will also cause serious injuries.

Every rep during each exercise should be smooth and controlled. We want to control the weight, not let the weight control *us.* If you're deciding to start a strength training program, I would suggest you do some research on how to perform the exercises the right way. *YouTube* is a great place to learn "how-to's".

Practice gym etiquette

Having poor gym etiquette is easily the biggest reason why people get the most grief. There is nothing more annoying than weights being left out and people hollering for no reason. Don't be *that* guy or girl.

The gym is a place where we should respect the equipment and also the people around us. Practicing gym etiquette is as simple as re-racking the weights you use and being aware of the people around you. This may seem very obvious and even unnecessary to bring up, but believe me, poor gym etiquette is an epidemic.

If you follow these two steps, you can be certain that you're practicing good gym etiquette.

2. High Intensity Interval Training

What is high intensity interval training? ACE Fitness' definition says,

> High Intensity Interval Training (HIIT) is a system of organizing cardiorespiratory training which calls for repeated bouts of short duration, high-intensity exercise intervals intermingled with periods of lower intensity intervals of active recovery. On a 1-10 scale of perceived exertion,

high intensity can be considered anything over an effort level of 7. When using max heart rate (MHR) as a guide, high intensity can be considered exercising above 80% of MHR.

Modes of HIIT can include outdoor activities such as running or cycling, or using equipment such as treadmills, elliptical runners, stair-climbers or stationary bikes. HIIT training calls for challenging work-rates such as sprints (whether on a bicycle or running) for short time frames lasting from thirty seconds to two minutes.

I've found that HIIT isn't very well known or even talked about by the average gym-goers and non- athletes. This is quite unfortunate for many reasons, but here are 4 examples of the great benefits that most people are missing out on.

Why is HIIT a good method of choice?

1. You can burn fat more effectively and for a longer period of time.
2. You will retain more of your muscle mass.
3. You can do HIIT *anywhere*.
4. You will save time.

Note: HIIT also provides many of the same perks that strength training does when it comes to overall health.

(1) Burn fat more effectively and for a longer period of time

Who wouldn't want a more effective way to lose that stubborn and unwanted fat?! The good news is, HIIT is definitely a great method of choice. Here's why: A study done by Jeffery W. King, of East Tennessee University, determined that the participants who followed an 8 week HIIT program lost 2% of body fat and their counterparts (who were doing only steady-paced cardio) lost 0% of body fat.

The study also found that those who participated in the HIIT program burned up to 100 extra calories per day. With HIIT you are not only burning calories while you workout, you're also burning calories while you are at rest. Therefore, giving you a more effective way to burn fat and for longer periods of time. This isn't the case with a steady-paced cardio approach.

(2) Retain more muscle mass

Do you recall what was said about muscle retention in the strength training section? I talked about the importance of retaining muscle mass while losing fat for the opportunity to look "toned" and have an "in-shape" physique. I also mentioned that having a steady-paced cardio approach, at best, will only dwindle you down to a smaller version of your current physique.

If we want a great physique, it is *so* important that we do all we can to retain as much muscle as possible while we're trying to lose fat. With HIIT this isn't a problem. We're performing short and intense bursts of energy that put a high performance demand on our muscles. Our bodies will recognize that our muscles are being put to good use. Thus allowing our energy to come from fat instead of tapping into muscle as fuel, like we would during a steady-paced cardio session. Retaining lean muscle mass will allow us to maintain our strength while also increasing our endurance.

(3) Do it anywhere

HIIT can be done literally anywhere. Do you have a yard? How about a local park, or maybe a local swimming pool? How about some extra space at home? You can even just stay at the gym and do it. There are many ways and many different exercises you can do for a HIIT workout. You could do sprints, hill sprints, jump rope, burpees, run stairs, sprints on a bike, jumping jacks, knee-ups, and the list goes on. As long as you have a fair amount of space, you can get in a solid workout.

A great example of this is when I was prepping for a physique competition back in 2014 (which I ended up not competing in due to personal reasons). I literally went to my local park, found a hill and sprinted the heck out of it twice a week. Through proper nutrition and smart training I was able to get down to 8% body fat and still had 5 weeks to go before I was supposed to compete.

I didn't use any fancy equipment, I just went out and found a hill. This doesn't have to be complicated and there certainly is no reason why you can't have similar results if you eat clean and train effectively.

So, get creative and have fun with this. Get outside, include your friends, make it a competition; what ever! You'll be happier than jogging on an indoor treadmill and you will most definitely be happier with your results.

(4) Save time

Most beginner HIIT programs that I've seen usually last about 15-20 minutes. Don't get me wrong, it is an intense 15-20 minutes, but guess what? That's way less than the average person will spend doing steady-paced cardio. We live busy lives in a fast paced world, which makes HIIT even more attractive because of its time efficiency.

3. Yoga

Before digging into it and learning the truth, my limited understanding of yoga was that I would have to wear tight pants and do flamboyant stretches. For a guy, that was a hard pill to swallow. However, I found that it's actually nothing like I once thought. Now I can honestly say I will never go a day without practicing yoga.

As it turns out, I learned that yoga is great for just about anything fitness related, and even better, I didn't have to wear tight yoga pants. Thank God.

I believe that yoga is the perfect puzzle piece to go along with strength training and HIIT. I've witnessed the positive effects of yoga not only in my own training, but in many of my peers' as well.

It is a great way to improve flexibility, endurance, subtle strength and poor posture. All of which play huge roles in achieving our fitness goals. The more flexible you are, the more strength you will have because your muscles can work more efficiently. The more endurance you have, the more effectively you can complete your HIIT. The more subtle strength you have, the better you can control the weights during strength training. The better your posture, the less likely you will be to get injured in the gym. You will also be less likely to have nagging back, shoulder or neck pains that will hinder you from even making it to the gym.

You see, everything is connected and yoga can be the knot that will tie it all together. I've found that just 10-15 minutes a day can make drastic changes and improvements in all the areas of fitness previously stated. I strongly encourage you to give yoga a shot!

Beginner's basic workout programs for weight loss and muscle growth included on the next page.

Beginners basic weight loss/muscle growth training programs combining Strength training, HIIT and Yoga

For weight loss:

Starting out with **3 days** of strength training per week, **2 days** of HIIT per week and **4-5 days** of yoga per week.

Day 1: Legs & Abs (quads, hamstrings, calves & abs)

- Squat: 4 sets X 12 reps (60-90 seconds rest between sets)

-Lying hamstring curl: 3 sets X 12 reps (45-60 seconds rest between sets)

-Leg extension: 3 sets X 12 reps (45-60 seconds rest between sets)

-Standing calf raise: 3 sets X 15 reps (45-60 seconds rest between sets)

-Leg raises in roman chair (abs): 3 sets X 15 reps (45-

60 seconds rest between sets)

*This workout should take approximately <u>60</u> minutes

<u>Day 2:</u> Push day (chest, shoulders & triceps followed by 20 minutes of HIIT)

-Incline dumbbell chest press: 4 sets X 10 reps (60-90 seconds rest between sets)

-Overhead dumbbell shoulder press: 3 sets X 10 reps (60-90 seconds rest between sets)

-Flat dumbbell chest fly: 3 sets X 12 reps (45-60 seconds rest between sets)

- Standing upright row: 3 sets X 12 reps (45-60 seconds rest between sets)

- Cable triceps extension: 3 sets X 12 reps (45-60 seconds rest between sets)

HIIT: (20 minutes) 3 rounds, 45 seconds high intensity, 15 seconds rest. Take 60 seconds recovery between rounds.

This workout can be done with any of the exercises listed in the HIIT section, so mix it up!

*This workout should take approximately 70 minutes

Day 3: Pull day (back, biceps & traps followed by 20 minutes of HIIT)

-Pull ups: Do as many sets as it takes to achieve 30 reps (if you cannot do pull ups, you can do lat pull downs: 3 sets X 12 reps) (45-60 seconds rest between sets)

-Deadlift: 4 sets X 10 reps (60-90 seconds rest between sets)

-Single arm dumbbell row: 3 sets X 12 reps each side (45-60 seconds rest between sets)

Alternating dumbbell curl: 4 sets X 10 reps each arm (45-60 seconds rest between sets)

Straight bar curl: 3 sets X 12 reps (45-60 seconds rest between sets)

HIIT: (20 minutes) 3 rounds, 45 seconds high intensity, 15 seconds rest. Take 60 seconds recovery between rounds.

This workout can be done with any of the exercises listed in the HIIT section, so mix it up!

*This workout should take approximately 70 minutes

Note: Yoga can be done on both rest days and training days given its low intensity. Aim for at least 10 minutes per day and for 4-5 days per week. I recommend attending a local yoga class or using an online instructor. You can find the best in the world at *doyouyoga.com* or on *YouTube.*

For muscle growth:

Starting out with **3 days** of strength training per week and **4-5 days** of yoga per week. (HIIT is not necessary for gaining muscle, but can be done **1-2 times** per week if you would like).

Note: This program will be very similar to the weight loss training program. This is because training is secondary to nutrition. In order to build muscle, you will need to be in a caloric surplus, as opposed to a caloric deficit when trying to lose weight. (See definitions: pg. 97)

Day 1: Legs & Abs (quads, hamstrings, calves & abs)

- Squat: 4 sets X 8-10 reps (60-90 seconds rest

between sets)

-Lying hamstring curl: 3 sets X 12 reps (45-60 seconds rest between sets)

-Leg extension: 3 sets X 12 reps (45-60 seconds rest between sets)

-Standing calf raise: 3 sets X 15 reps (45-60 seconds rest between sets)

-Leg raises in roman chair (abs): 3 sets X 15 reps (45-60 seconds rest between sets)

*This workout should take approximately <u>60</u> minutes

<u>Day 2</u>: Push day (chest, shoulders & triceps)

-Incline dumbbell chest press: 4 sets X 10 reps (60-90 seconds rest between sets)

-Overhead dumbbell shoulder press: 4 sets X 10 reps (60-90 seconds rest between sets)

-Flat dumbbell chest fly: 4 sets X 12 reps (45-60 seconds rest between sets)

- Standing upright row: 4 sets X 12 reps (45-60

seconds rest between sets)

- Cable triceps extension: 3 sets X 12 reps (45-60 seconds rest between sets)

*This workout should take approximately <u>60</u> minutes

<u>Day 3:</u> Pull day (back, biceps & traps)

-Pull ups: Do as many sets as it takes to achieve 30 reps (if you cannot do pull ups, you can do lat pull downs: 4 sets X 10 reps) (45-60 seconds rest between sets)

-Deadlift: 4 sets X 8-10 reps (60-90 seconds rest between sets)

-Single arm dumbbell row: 4 sets X 10 reps each side (45-60 seconds rest between sets)

Alternating dumbbell curl: 4 sets X 10 reps each arm (45-60 seconds rest between sets)

Straight bar curl: 4 sets X 12 reps (45-60 seconds rest between sets)

*This workout should take approximately <u>60</u> minutes

Note: Yoga can be done on both rest days and training days given its low intensity. Aim for at least 10 minutes per day and for 4-5 days per week. I recommend attending a local yoga class or using an online instructor. You can find the best in the world at *doyouyoga.com* or on *YouTube.*

If you would like to add in one or two HIIT workouts per week, you certainly can.

HIIT: (20 minutes) 3 rounds, 45 seconds high intensity, 15 seconds rest. Take 60 seconds recovery between rounds.

This workout can be done with any of the exercises listed in the HIIT section, so mix it up!

If you are unsure on how to do any of the exercises listed, make sure you either ask someone who knows what they're doing, or look online to learn the proper form and execution of the movement. Also, if you feel that either of these programs become too easy, please move on to a more difficult program. Progression is key.

These basic programs will only get you

so far and they are only meant to start you off on the right track. Once you are ready to move on from these programs, I encourage you to look online and do some research on intermediate strength training, HIIT and yoga programs to find out which one will best suit you and your goals.

6 REST DAYS ARE THE BEST DAYS

"The most important day in any running program is rest. Rest days give your muscles time to recover so you can run again. Your muscles build in strength as you rest."

-Hal Higdon: American writer and former marathon runner

A mindset that many people have when it comes to hitting fitness goals is, "the more work that I do in the gym, the better off I'll be." I thought the same thing. I thought that if I went to the gym 7 days a week and worked out for 2 hours then I would get better results than the person who goes 4 days a week and only works out for 1 hour. I was looking at it strictly as a numbers game; more effort equals more results, right? Not always.

The key to getting the best results is giving your body the amount of rest that it needs to properly recover from the butt whooping you gave it in the gym. It's all about working smarter, not harder. When I grasped this concept I noticed a huge difference in my energy levels and the quality of my workouts. I don't feel fatigued and tired, rather, I feel refreshed both before and after my training. It's no doubt that taking more rest days has been the reason that my body's response has been drastically different.

How many days per week should I be at the gym?

This is a question that often comes up

when talking about fitness. In my opinion, if you're just starting out, there is nothing wrong with training only 2-3 times per week. Your body has an adjustment period that it will need to go through. It will need to get used to being more active, especially if you have little-to-no experience with exercising. Less frequency in the beginning will allow for these things to happen without risking injury or burning yourself out too quickly. You're making lifestyle changes and if you go too hard right from the start, you will run the risk of overwhelming both your body and your mindset.

This is a journey, not a quick-fix.

Make sleep a priority

Since we're on the topic of rest, I think it's necessary that we address how important sleeping actually is. You've probably heard people say something like, "make sure you get your 8 hours tonight", right? But in reality, how many of us are actually making it a priority? I've heard friends say things like "Nahh, I'll sleep when I'm dead." Don't get me wrong, I definitely respect the hustle, but this mindset doesn't do us any favors, especially when we're trying to achieve our health and fitness goals. It is when we are sleeping that our bodies do the most repair from our workouts and other daily tasks.

When we are asleep, our bodies are also releasing growth hormone. Growth hormone isn't only for building big muscles, it has many other benefits, such as: promoting fat-loss, lowering fat storage, raising calcium retention (for stronger bones), boosting the immune system and helping our organs function smoothly.

There are plenty additional benefits from getting the right amount of sleep. From this one example of growth hormone, you can see that sleep is most definitely an important factor in reaching our goals.

To get the most benefit from your sleep is to make sure that it is *quality* sleep. But, everyone is different, so the amount of hours you need may be different than the next person. Check out this link from the National Sleep Foundation to see how many hours their scientists recommend for you!

https://sleepfoundation.org/sites/default/fil es/STREPchanges_1.png

If you have trouble sleeping or you feel that you sleep too light, try out a high quality melatonin supplement. (Follow the recommendations from chapter 3 on how to choose the right brand of supplement). This will allow you to get into the deeper REM (rapid eye movement) cycles throughout the night and ensure that you get quality sleep.

7 NINETY DAYS TO LIFE CHANGE

"A goal without a plan is just a wish."

-Antoine de Saint-Exupery: French writer, poet, and pioneering aviator

The difference between people who achieve their goals and the people who don't, begins with the tip of a pen. The ones who write down their goals and look back on them regularly are more likely to succeed at what they are trying to accomplish. They are telling their subconscious minds that they have a plan and they're willing to do whatever it takes to get it done. The subconscious mind is a very powerful tool that we can learn to control if we take the right steps.

If you and I were talking about health and fitness goals, this is the advice I would give. Pick a goal and give it some urgency. This could be something like running a 5K, doing a fitness competition and even wanting to slim down for a high school reunion or attending a friend's wedding. Whatever relates to your specific desires, choose it and make sure it is something that will push you. Set a 90-day deadline for this goal, and then - here's the fun part - tell the world.

I learned this at a workshop event I attended in Chicago. The speaker gave a simple formula for achieving goals more effectively. He said: "Say yes, tell the world, and figure it out. After completing steps one through three, you plan it, you do it, and you review it. Rinse and repeat."

Once we get ourselves out of our comfort zone and announce our goal to our friends, co-workers, family and others, we don't want to look like we lack commitment. So what does this added pressure do for us? It pushes us to work extra hard so we don't have to deal with people giving us grief about not accomplishing what we set out to do. It sparks a sense of urgency in us and all of a sudden we start picking up some momentum - we start figuring it out and creating new habits.

Skipping the gym no longer becomes a regular occurrence. Throwing in an extra cheat meal because it's "just *one* bowl of ice cream" doesn't happen anymore because suddenly, each day matters.

You only have 90 days now; one of those days where you "mess up" is one-ninetieth of the time that you have left. There is no time on the back end to make up for mistakes. Do you see what I'm saying? We can't just aim for "someday" goals because "someday" never comes if we don't discipline ourselves.

We then must continue to plan, do, and review throughout the process. Apply the things you learn in this book and you will be amazed at the life changes you can achieve in 90 days.

8 DON'T QUIT BEFORE THE CLAY GETS WARM

I remember early on when I first got into training I came across a fitness icon that I had never heard of before. His name is Greg Plitt, and he is someone that I've looked up to ever since. He was such a fiery and passionate person and it allowed for his viewers to really connect with him. He has since passed from a freak accident, but his words will forever have a lasting impact on not only myself, but the entire fitness industry.

He made a video that changed the way I looked at exercising, goal setting, and everything in between. It changed the way that I looked at life in general. He basically punched me in the gut through the computer screen because his words were so true and they really made me think and dig deeper. If you're serious about hitting your goals; I highly recommend you watch it. It is called "Keeping the fire alive by Greg Plitt" and can be found on *YouTube*. Disclaimer: He says quite a few curse words, but if you can look past that, this video will rock your world in the best way possible.

In the video he uses an analogy that I think is absolutely perfect and relevant to all of us who go to the gym seeking better health and fitness. Rather than me trying to explain it, here is his exact quote.

The scenario I always talk about is cold clay. In the movie Ghost, Demi Moore is making a pot right; she grabs a piece of clay. Imagine that being a metaphor, being your body right? For 20 years, 30 years, 40 years it's been sitting there on the shelf just cold, not moving, lethargic, no energy, and no motion at all. You put it on the wheel, start spinning it, you grab some water and you try to shape it but it's not moving, man. It's not moving at all.

But as you start to get your hands moving you start heating it up heating it up heating it up. That's your body going to the gym. Week after week, week after week, week after week and then all of a sudden BOOM! It starts moving. All of a sudden you start creating something. But before you couldn't. And then when you create what you want you let it dry and cool off, and then bam, it's locked. It's not going anywhere.

What I'm trying to say is that the transformation portion is ten times, a hundred times harder than actually being in shape. Maintaining an in-shape state is simple, guys. It's transforming that is so hard. But that makes the transform stage and being in shape SO DESIRABLE. 'Cause it's so freaking hard to transform it.

-Greg Plitt

Remember, this is a journey, friends.
Don't quit before the clay gets warm.

9 THE CHOICE IS YOURS

"You miss 100% of the shots you don't take."

-Wayne Gretzky: Hockey hall of famer, 4 time Stanley Cup champion, known as "the greatest hockey player of all time"

As the quote above says, you will miss 100% of the shots you don't take. This isn't only relevant in sports, it is relevant in every day life and it is certainly relevant in your fitness journey. We've come to the end and you're about to finish reading this book. So the question is, are you going to take a shot?

A shot at creating a better life for yourself? A shot at your goals? A shot at feeling better? A shot at your ideal physique? A shot at optimal health? The choice is yours. I sincerely hope that the words and the practical steps stated in this book have inspired you to begin your journey towards health and fitness. But even more importantly, I hope that you follow through with it.

I hope that you get to experience what it feels like to transform yourself through hard work and dedication. Don't just be inspired, rather instead, be inspired *and* be willing to take action. Couple the two together and you will be unstoppable.

What has been holding you back up until this point? What may be stopping you right now? You may feel like you can't do it, you can't reach your goal physique, or you can't stay dedicated to the hard work that this journey entails. What ever it is that the little voice inside your head is telling you, politely tell it to shut up, because you, yes you, can absolutely do this. Just make the decision and follow through.

ACTION STEPS

"I've always believed that if you put in the work, the results will come. I don't do things half-heartedly. Because I know if I do, I can expect half-hearted results."

-Michael Jordan: NBA hall of famer, 6 time NBA champion

At the beginning of this book I told you that I would give you the basic tools that you would need to start your journey toward health and fitness. I also mentioned that none of these things would matter unless *you* put them into action. I held up my end of the bargain, now I ask you to hold up your end.

Your goals are waiting for you and the only thing that can stop you is *you*. So what do you do next? You've read this book, now you have to apply it. I want to leave you with four action steps that you can apply as soon as you close this book.

1. Just say YES

- Say YES to a new lifestyle.

- Say YES to achieving your goals.

- Commit yourself now and you will thank yourself later.

- Write out your *"why"* and 90 day goal in the pages provided at the end of this book. (pgs. 104-107)

- Tell someone you're close to what your goals are and ask them to hold you accountable.

2. Go find a gym that you like and sign up

- Some gyms cost as little as $10 per month.

- You will be surrounded by like-minded individuals who are on the same journey.

3. Find a partner

- I'm sure you have a friend or relative that would like to get healthy as well.

- Accountability is huge.

- You don't have to be in this alone.

4. Take it seriously

- Nobody has ever achieved anything great by putting in 60, 70, 80 or even 90% of their effort. Be all-in and give this 100%.

- Fight for your goals and be consistent.

- Take the time to build good habits that are going to push you closer to your goals.

Thank you so much for reading! I'd love to connect with you on social media!

@jordandunham_

facebook.com/Jordan.dunham.98

I would also like to give a special shout-out to a few key people who helped me with creating this book. I appreciate you and your hard work more than I could ever say. Thank you! :)

Melissa Yang – Editing & Proofing

Igor Kasyanyuk – Photography

Matt Yang – Front & Back Cover Design

Quick definitions to become familiar with:

Accessory movements: Exercises that use only one joint or muscle group at a time (bicep curls, triceps extensions, hamstring curls and quad extensions are examples)

Antioxidants: Stops the oxidation process that is continuously happening inside and outside of the body

Blood sugar: The concentration of glucose in the blood

Calories: Energy from food that fuels the body

Caloric deficit: A shortage in the amount of calories consumed relative to the amount of calories required for maintenance of current body weight (resulting in weight loss)

Caloric surplus: An increase in the amount of calories consumed relative to the amount of calories required for maintenance of current body weight (resulting in weight gain)

<u>Carbohydrates:</u> Provide fuel and energy during exercise and spares protein to preserve muscle during exercise

<u>Compound movements:</u> Exercises that involve more than one joint or muscle group at a time (deadlifts, bench press, squats and overhead press are examples)

<u>Drop sets:</u> A technique for continuing an exercise with a lower weight once muscle failure has been achieved at a higher weight

<u>Fat:</u> Reserves energy, protects vital organs and transfers fat-soluble vitamins

<u>Glycemic Index:</u> A system that ranks food 1-100 based on their effect on blood-sugar levels

<u>Glycemic rollercoaster:</u> The up and down process of blood-sugar and insulin levels due to a poor food plan

Gym etiquette: Respecting the equipment in the gym and the people around you

High glycemic: Food that is ranked 70 and higher on the glycemic index chart

HIIT: A system of organizing cardiorespiratory training which calls for repeated bouts of short duration, high-intensity exercise intervals intermingled with periods of lower intensity intervals of active recovery.

Insulin: A hormone that regulates the amount of glucose in the blood

Lean body mass: The total body weight minus the body fat (typically around 60-90% of total body weight)

Low glycemic: Food that is ranked 55 and below on the glycemic index chart

Macronutrients: The nutrients that provide calories (Carbohydrates, proteins and fats)

Meal replacement shakes: A complete, balanced and healthy meal in shake form

Micronutrients: The nutrients required to manage physiological functions (vitamins, minerals and antioxidants)

Minerals: Contains essential nutrients needed to survive and carry out daily functions

Nutrition: The process of eating the right foods in order to grow and be healthy

Oxidation: Any chemical reaction that involves the moving of electrons

Progressive overload: The gradual increase of stress placed upon the body during exercise training

Proper form: The correct and safe way to effectively perform a certain exercise

Protein: Necessary for the structure, function and regulation of the body's tissues and organs

RDA levels: The estimated amount of nutrients needed per day in order to remain healthy (equivalent to aiming for a D- in math class)

Reps: The number of times within a "set" that a specific exercise is performed

Rest days: Days taken off from the gym in order for the body to rest, recover and re-build

Rest periods: The time spent resting and recovering in between sets

Sets: The cycles of reps completed

Static Stretching: stretches that are held in a challenging position for an extended period of time

Strength training: a type of physical exercise specializing in the use of resistance to induce muscular contraction which builds strength, anaerobic endurance, and size of skeletal muscles

<u>Supersets:</u> Combining two exercises together into one set

<u>Supplementation:</u> A way to help fill the nutrition gaps that many people are missing

<u>Tempo:</u> The speed and pace at which an exercise is performed

<u>Vitamins:</u> Allows the body to break down and use the basic elements and energy that food provides

<u>Warming-up:</u> a gradual increase in intensity in physical activity followed by a more intense workout

<u>Whole foods:</u> Food that is considered healthy because it is grown naturally, has not been processed, and contains no artificial ingredients

<u>Working sets:</u> The sets within a routine that are meant to do the actual work (as opposed to warm up sets)

<u>Yoga:</u> A spiritual and ascetic discipline, a part of which, including breath control, simple meditation, and the adoption of specific bodily postures, is widely practiced for health and relaxation

What is your "Why?" Use this section to write it out. Be specific!

_____

_____

_____

_____

_____

_____

_____

_____

_____

_____

_____

_____

_____

_____

_____

_____

_____

_____

_____

_____

_____

What is your 90 day goal? Use this section to write it out. Be specific!

_____

_____

_____

_____

_____

_____

_____

_____

_____

_____

_____

_____

_____

_____

_____

_____

_____

_____

_____

_____

_____

Workout - Progression Tracker

Remember, progression is key in achieving your goals. Use this tracker to write down and keep record of your gym sessions. Each time you workout look back on your previous training sessions and aim to progress. Small increments of forward progression is the goal here!

Example:

Let's say you trained legs last Monday. The next Monday rolls around and it's time to train them again. Before you begin, take a look back at the records you wrote down of your previous leg workout and analyze what those numbers are. (Writing space provided on pages to come).

To keep it simple, we'll hypothetically say that you accomplished **4 sets** of **12 reps** on squats using **100 pounds**, and you did them relatively easy. This is a sign that the weight is becoming too light and you need to add more in order to continue breaking down the muscle fibers. Remember, this is what causes growth.

When you look back and see that you accomplished the recommended sets and reps with whatever weight you used, aim to add at least 5 pounds to the bar and accomplish those same sets and reps. (This strategy can be used with any exercise). In this example, this would mean that you now accomplished **4 sets** of **12 reps** with **105 pounds**. 5 more pounds than you did last week. Enter, progression.

Always be on the hunt for progression, but also remember to keep strict form. There may be times where you increase the weight in certain exercises and you fail to hit the recommended number of sets and reps. This is okay, just use the same weight until you achieve the number of sets and reps that you are aiming to hit. Do not force yourself into sloppy form just to hit numbers. This will not help you in the long run. Also note: if you are hitting sets and reps that are significantly lower than your target, lower the weight. This shows that you've added too much too soon. To sum everything up, just listen to your body. If it's telling you that a 5 pound increase isn't enough, or it's too much, increase or decrease the weight based on how it felt while you were performing the exercise.

Continue following this method, along with the other things you've learned in this book and you will see your strength and overall progress sky-rocket.

Track your progress on pages 113-119!

<u>Note:</u> Feel free to use these same templates when you move onto intermediate and advanced workout plans. I also recommend making copies of these templates so you can continue tracking your progress outside of this book.

Example of how to use the tracker on pg. 112.

LIGHTING THE FIRE

Exercise	Sets & Reps Target	Set	# of Reps Achieved	Weight Being Used	Target Reps Achieved?	Next Week's Weight
Squats	4 Sets X 12 Reps	1 2 3 4	X 12 X 12 X 12 X 12	100 Pounds	YES!	105 Pounds
Lying Hamstring Curls	3 Sets X 12 Reps	1 2 3	X 12 X 12 X (10)	50 Pounds	X Not Quite	50 Pounds
		1 2 3 4	X X X X			
		1 2 3 4	X X X X			
		1 2 3 4	X X X X			
		1 2 3 4	X X X X			
		1 2 3 4	X X X X			
		1 2 3 4	X X X X			
		1 2 3 4	X X X X			

Exercise	Sets & Reps Target	Set	# of Reps Achieved	Weight Being Used	Target Reps Achieved?	Next Week's Weight
		1	X			
		2	X			
		3	X			
		4	X			
		1	X			
		2	X			
		3	X			
		4	X			
		1	X			
		2	X			
		3	X			
		4	X			
		1	X			
		2	X			
		3	X			
		4	X			
		1	X			
		2	X			
		3	X			
		4	X			
		1	X			
		2	X			
		3	X			
		4	X			
		1	X			
		2	X			
		3	X			
		4	X			
		1	X			
		2	X			
		3	X			
		4	X			
		1	X			
		2	X			
		3	X			
		4	X			

Exercise	Sets & Reps Target	Set	# of Reps Achieved	Weight Being Used	Target Reps Achieved?	Next Week's Weight
		1 2 3 4	X X X X			
		1 2 3 4	X X X X			
		1 2 3 4	X X X X			
		1 2 3 4	X X X X			
		1 2 3 4	X X X X			
		1 2 3 4	X X X X			
		1 2 3 4	X X X X			
		1 2 3 4	X X X X			
		1 2 3 4	X X X X			

Exercise	Sets & Reps Target	Set	# of Reps Achieved	Weight Being Used	Target Reps Achieved?	Next Week's Weight
		1	X			
		2	X			
		3	X			
		4	X			
		1	X			
		2	X			
		3	X			
		4	X			
		1	X			
		2	X			
		3	X			
		4	X			
		1	X			
		2	X			
		3	X			
		4	X			
		1	X			
		2	X			
		3	X			
		4	X			
		1	X			
		2	X			
		3	X			
		4	X			
		1	X			
		2	X			
		3	X			
		4	X			
		1	X			
		2	X			
		3	X			
		4	X			
		1	X			
		2	X			
		3	X			
		4	X			

Exercise	Sets & Reps Target	Set	# of Reps Achieved	Weight Being Used	Target Reps Achieved?	Next Week's Weight
		1	X			
		2	X			
		3	X			
		4	X			
		1	X			
		2	X			
		3	X			
		4	X			
		1	X			
		2	X			
		3	X			
		4	X			
		1	X			
		2	X			
		3	X			
		4	X			
		1	X			
		2	X			
		3	X			
		4	X			
		1	X			
		2	X			
		3	X			
		4	X			
		1	X			
		2	X			
		3	X			
		4	X			
		1	X			
		2	X			
		3	X			
		4	X			
		1	X			
		2	X			
		3	X			
		4	X			

Exercise	Sets & Reps Target	Set	# of Reps Achieved	Weight Being Used	Target Reps Achieved?	Next Week's Weight
		1	X			
		2	X			
		3	X			
		4	X			
		1	X			
		2	X			
		3	X			
		4	X			
		1	X			
		2	X			
		3	X			
		4	X			
		1	X			
		2	X			
		3	X			
		4	X			
		1	X			
		2	X			
		3	X			
		4	X			
		1	X			
		2	X			
		3	X			
		4	X			
		1	X			
		2	X			
		3	X			
		4	X			
		1	X			
		2	X			
		3	X			
		4	X			
		1	X			
		2	X			
		3	X			
		4	X			

Exercise	Sets & Reps Target	Set	# of Reps Achieved	Weight Being Used	Target Reps Achieved?	Next Week's Weight
		1	X			
		2	X			
		3	X			
		4	X			
		1	X			
		2	X			
		3	X			
		4	X			
		1	X			
		2	X			
		3	X			
		4	X			
		1	X			
		2	X			
		3	X			
		4	X			
		1	X			
		2	X			
		3	X			
		4	X			
		1	X			
		2	X			
		3	X			
		4	X			
		1	X			
		2	X			
		3	X			
		4	X			
		1	X			
		2	X			
		3	X			
		4	X			
		1	X			
		2	X			
		3	X			
		4	X			

Exercise	Sets & Reps Target	Set	# of Reps Achieved	Weight Being Used	Target Reps Achieved?	Next Week's Weight
		1	X			
		2	X			
		3	X			
		4	X			
		1	X			
		2	X			
		3	X			
		4	X			
		1	X			
		2	X			
		3	X			
		4	X			
		1	X			
		2	X			
		3	X			
		4	X			
		1	X			
		2	X			
		3	X			
		4	X			
		1	X			
		2	X			
		3	X			
		4	X			
		1	X			
		2	X			
		3	X			
		4	X			
		1	X			
		2	X			
		3	X			
		4	X			
		1	X			
		2	X			
		3	X			
		4	X			

JORDAN PAUL DUNHAM

LIGHTING THE FIRE